LADIES GUIDE TO FASTING:

A lead to shed fat, build hormonal stability and improve energy

By

Mary M. Bennett

Table of content

Introduction

We have never needed another worldview for well-being. In the past couple of years, constant circumstances like Alzheimer's, malignant growth, diabetes, infertility, autoimmunity, temperament jumble, cardiovascular sickness, and, surprisingly, persistent agony have soared. What may be the most dampening about this flood is that large numbers of these findings are occurring to ladies. However ladies are as yet given a one-size-fits-all arrangement that seldom considers their hormonal requirements, leaving them feeling unheard, out of replies, and, the majority of all, still wiped out.

We as a whole have minutes we think back on and understand that in a moment our life was changed for eternity. It is urgent to know that when your well-being goes to pieces, you want only one individual to accept and give you trust.

Transforming one's eating routine is an effective method for beginning, all food varieties are not will be not made equivalent since some foods develop your well-being while some drain you.

You were astonished at how great your body will answer changing your eating regimen to quality food that will assist with building your framework.

Fasting, assists with each part of metabolic well-being, from weight reduction and hypertension to insulin opposition, irritation, and bringing down cholesterol. there is likewise logical proof that fasting fixes our stomach microbiome, further develops neurodegenerative illnesses like dementia and Alzheimer's, reboots a striving insusceptible framework, and can control up satisfaction synapses like dopamine, serotonin, and GABA.

While logical proof is clear is fasting recuperates, there exists a tremendous bling spot: A one-size-fits-all way to deal with fasting doesn't work, particularly for ladies. However invigorating as more individuals may be integrating irregular fasting into their way of life, three inquiries have arisen that are not being tended to.

The first is how long would it be advisable for one to quick?

Irregular fasting is considered going 13 to 15 hours without food. In the interim, one of the most renowned fasting concentrates on uncovering that a three-day quick can dispense with precancerous cells and reboot your entire safe framework. As these logical articles become more standard, and fasting becomes more famous, a great deal of sentiments are being thrown around on lengthy an individual ought to quick. This makes it extraordinarily confounding for some to decide how long they ought to quit.

The subsequent inquiry is, what food is best matched with fasting?

Fasting specialists have been zeroing in on the recuperating that occurs inside the fasting window, leaving fasting in obscurity concerning the mending significance of food when they do eat. Food ought not to be forgotten about, when you pair the right food varieties with fasting, wonder happens, particularly for ladies.

The third and most significant inquiry is, do ladies have to be quick uniquely in contrast to men?

Ladies are profoundly impacted by the month-to-month and menopausal swings of chemicals. The complexities of our sex chemicals oestrogen, progesterone, and testosterone - expect that we focus harder on spikes of cortisol and insulin that can occur with an expansion in stress, exercise, food, and fasting also. At the point when we use fasting to flip our metabolic switch, we want to adjust it with our hormones.

Even though men are hormonally driven too, their own are not as delicate to these spikes. For a lady to understand the full medical advantages of fasting, she has to know when and how to flip her metabolic switch as per her hormonal cycles.

If a lady chooses too quickly and doesn't match up that quickly with her period, unfriendly side effects might show up, for example, rashes, hair loss, anxiety, missed feminine cycle thyroid issues, and issues with resting. These are side effects that can be stayed away from when a lady figures out how to quick for her special body. Done appropriately, fasting can determine many circumstances ladies are battling with. The equivalent goes for menopausal ladies who may never again have a cycle yet have hormonal necessities.

On the whole, this book will be a guide to light as you figure out how to utilise fasting and assume back command over your well-being.

Chapter 1

It's not your issue

Your body is an almost wonderful machine. It comprises more than 30 trillion cells that behave like a bound-together group, striving to ensure you flourish. Every individual cell resembles a little industrial facility that produces energy by consuming fat, processing glucose, and assembling cell reinforcements. These cells know when to drive you up with energy so you can play out an undertaking, and when to call you back so you can rest. At the point when you eat, they gobble up the supplement you have accommodated them and utilise those supplements to do the errands expected to keep you working at your best. If food isn't accessible, they switch over to an elective fuel source to guarantee you have the strength and mental lucidity to work. At the point when receptors outwardly of these cells sense chemicals flowing in your blood, they open up their door and let these chemicals in. They proficiently adjust to any physical, substance, or close-to-home impacts that you toss in their direction.

Here is the test: they need your help, they need specific supplements to work appropriately as supplements such as great fat, amino acids, minerals, and nutrients. At the point when they don't get support, they quit having the option to go about their business. There are five manners by which diets have driven you down a twisty way, one that you can course-address whenever. I refer to it as "the five fizzled" and they incorporate, calorie limitation, unfortunate food quality, consistent cortisol floods, expanding poisonous burdens, and one-size-fits-all methodologies.When you comprehend these eating regimen disappointments, you will see that you have been on a hell of a well-being thrill ride. Most eating regimens have aimlessly detached you from your body's configuration, driving you straight into the arms of dissatisfaction, self-uncertainty, and doubt with your body. The outcome you need can happen when you move back from the requirements of this diet culture, understand how astounding your body was planned, and embrace another well-being worldview that works with the mind-blowing female body you get to live in.

Know that mending starts when you can excuse yourself for the past. As you go through these five disappointments, realise that there is a decent opportunity that not your shortcomings or past eating regimen hasn't worked for you. Relinquishing such bad contemplations will serve you as you step into this new better adaptation of yourself.

The bombed five
1. The calorie limitation abstains from food
Assuming there is one fantasy I could separate from your brain, it would be that counting calories keeps you slim. You have imagined that eating less and practising more will give you enduring well-being and more satisfaction.

Each time you eat less and practise more, you change your metabolic set point. Your set point is where your body keeps up with its weight inside a favoured scope of calories. Whenever you return to eating more and working out less, the pounds do return exceptionally simple since you are over your set point.

2. Unfortunate food quality decisions
At the point when you see a low-fat level on an item, immediately set it back on the rack. Liken low fat to high sugar, high poisonous fixing two things that will rapidly make you pack on the pounds. For what reason did these new stylish low-fat food items

make you put on weight? The incongruity is that we are currently finding that ultra-handled food sources, similar to those found in numerous famous eating regimens, make us insulin-safe. This is a term that is getting a part of the press nowadays, generally because countless individuals are battling with weight and diabetes. Insulin opposition is a condition where your cells can never again effectively use insulin as a chemical to accompany the sugar from your food into your cells. At the point when your cells become unfit to involve glucose for fuel, not only will you experience an exhaustion in energy but they will store the unused glucose as fat.

How is insulin intended to function?

Insulin is your sugar-putting away chemical. Your pancreas delivers this chemical after you eat dinner to accompany the sugar from that feast into your cells. The more sugar thick a dinner, the more prominent the insulin delivery. A consistent motion of insulin will flood your cells, overpowering the receptor locales that permit the chemicals to play out their work. Receptor destinations are the entryways outwardly of our cells that open up to give chemicals access. The more insulin floods these doors, the more blocked these entryways become like major cell traffic. It is as of now that your cells become hard of hearing to insulin.

3. Spiking cortisol floods

This is the foe of insulin. You can't be in that frame of mind of pressure and construct well-being simultaneously. At the point when cortisol goes up, so does insulin. How can it function? How about we return to the calorie limitation and consume fewer calories than you might have attempted before? The unbending nature of these eating regimens frequently creates pressure, spiking your cortisol levels. You begin decreasing the quantity of calories you eat, which makes you ravenous and bad-tempered. This new disturbed state makes a battle or battle response in your mind, and your cerebrum answers by delivering cortisol into your circulatory system, letting your body know there is a current emergency. Your body answers this emergency signal by closing down processing, ending fat consumption, and raising your glucose levels so you are ready to deal with this upsetting circumstance. As your glucose levels go up, insulin ascends to fulfil the new sugar needs. Again, a flood of insulin overpowers your cells. The insane part is that all of this occurs without a solitary snack of food entering your mouth.

Dreary cortisol spikes will obstruct your counting calories results. Any unbending eating routine that you need to reliably muscle your direction through will save cortisol for a long time. However, cortisol spikes don't simply happen because your supervisor over-burdens you with work, or you have a contention with your life partner. Frequently cortisol spikes can happen when you bounce on a careful nutritional plan that is prohibitive and difficult to squeeze into your way of life.

It can likewise rise when you are overexercising, attempting to compel your body into a condition of well-being.

4. Openness to Poisonous fixings

Poisons make you fat. At the point when you investigate a mirror and reveal the difficult weight that will not disappear; reevaluate the reason for that fat. It's not there to worry you, your body didn't in a real sense, have any idea how to separate the substance in your food, so it puts it in your fat stores so it wouldn't hurt the organs that keep you alive. It's a splendid framework your body has made for your drawn-out endurance.

5. One-size-fits-all methodologies

There is nobody ideal eating routine for everybody, we as a whole have different hormonal necessities at various seasons of our lives, and our eating regimen needs to oblige that rhythmic movement. Perhaps of the greatest mischief that has at any point been finished to ladies' wellbeing is the interminable conviction that we as a whole ought to be on a similar eating regimen. Every single one of your sex chemicals has different food prerequisites. This implies you want to change the food you eat to match the back-and-forth movement of your chemicals. If you are a reusing lady most eating regimens make them eat the same way the entire month, potentially neutralising the necessities of your hormones, if a postmenopausal lady with low hormonal creation, slims down are not outfitted towards giving you food arrangements that boost your age suitable chemical creation. The eating regimen you are probably going to have is organised with a one-size-fits-all methodology.

As you step into a worldview, I need to call attention to one or other spot where this one-size-fits-all approach annihilates us. Its examination, remarkably, correlated with one another. Rather than attempting to make our own delightful special well-being way, we watch different ladies and the outcomes they get with their eating regimens and expect our bodies can accomplish a similar outcome.

Over and over again we decide our self-esteem by contrasting ourselves with another lady's feature reel. This is as harmful to our bodies as any of the five bombed diet techniques recorded. Remember that even though we are living in a female body, we don't all have a similar way of life needs. Each lady is her exceptional hormonal excursion. Finding an eating routine that is modified to our chemicals is urgent if we have any desire to prevail in our well-being.

Chapter 2

The recuperating force of fasting

In the fasting state, the body will scour for dead cells, harmed tissues, greasy stores, growths, and abscesses, which are all signed for fuel or ousted as waste. The end of these hindrances reestablishes the invulnerable framework usefulness and metabolic interaction to an ideal state.

On the off chance that somebody let you know there was a pill that could be useful to you look and feel more youthful, monitor stomach fat, and diminish the gamble of diabetes, malignant growth, and coronary illness, you'd be enticed to take it, couldn't you? Unfortunately, there's no such sorcery pill, be that as it may, brief times of fasting can assist you with accomplishing this, without the unsavoury after effects.

The bringing together hypothesis is that fasting serves to de-stress the body. By offering your body a reprieve to get up to speed with everything it isn't able to do when it's in the middle of processing and handling food, you might accomplish medical advantages. My methodology on withdrawals is to direct individuals through a 'block quick' - various consecutive days when the body is in a sped-up mending state, trailed by customised discontinuous fasting conventions to use as a component of a sound way of life or weight reduction plan. My form of block diets uses vegetable juices, stocks, and stomach wellbeing supporters instead of water-based diets which are a lot harder on the body and can exhaust supplement levels. Numerous monetarily accessible juices are just too high in sugar, and do not address the sustenance of the stomach microbes, crucial to accomplishing well-being results.

Underneath you'll find a short clarification of how fasting is remembered to apply its wellbeing impacts overall around the body, upheld by logical exploration.

How does fasting influence blood glucose control?
Fasting gainfully affects blood glucose control. At the end of another fasting test north of about fourteen days, insulin-intercepted glucose take-up rates expanded. On overweight ladies, the people who were limited to 500 calories consistently a day (with typical dietary in the middle between) showed lower fasting insulin levels and less insulin opposition than those on a standard calorie-

controlled diet. Notwithstanding, when individuals ate just a single feast a day at night for quite some time, it appeared to take more time for their insulin levels to increase in light of a morning glucose load.

Who needs to live for eternity?
(Indeed, for an additional 40 years)
We should check out one more chemical with a fundamentally the same as the design insulin. It's so comparable, it's known as insulin-like development factor, or IGF-1. IGF-1 has both positive and adverse consequences. Like insulin, it is anabolic, implying that it advises our cells to develop. If IGF-1 is kept high, our cells are continually partitioning and duplicating - great assuming we're attempting to assemble large muscles; not very great on the off chance that those cells become harmed and destructive. Elevated degrees of IGF-1 have been connected to prostate malignant growth and postmenopausal bosom disease. At the point when IGF-1 levels drop, the body eases back the creation of new cells and starts fixing old ones - DNA harm is bound to sort out. Fortunately fasting additionally decreases levels of IGF-1. At the point when the gathering of researchers in California hereditarily designed mice to have low degrees of IGF-1, they

found that they lived 40% longer. It chips away at individuals too. a gathering in a distant district of Ecuador who have low degrees of IGF-1 appear to be 'safe' to diabetes and malignant growth, despite having an exceptionally undesirable way of life. Nonetheless, not something can be packaged, not yet at any rate. The Ecadorians who have exhibited this incredible insusceptibility have a pre-existing condition called Laron Disorder Laron Condition accompanies development issues, so it isn't the enchanted response.

The main way you can normally decrease levels of IGF-1 is by fasting. In something like 24 hours of fasting, IGF falls. Fasting for three or four days, or slicing protein admission to beneath 0.95g/kg body weight/day, are the most effective ways to return IGF-1 to normal.

Fasting allows your body to have a spring-clean
Fasting turns on a significant interaction, called autophagy. The term autophagy signifies 'self-eating' and depicts the way that cells become empowered to distinguish and dispose of harmed or flawed parts. For instance, when a cell's energy force to be reckoned with the mitochondria becomes harmed they increment oxidative pressure, escalating the

pace of cell harm. This is much the same as power stations pouring out contamination. Autophagy empowers the cells to dispose of the defective mitochondria, permitting them to be supplanted by more 'energy effective' new ones. It likewise assists the body with battling diseases and recuperating from wounds. Autophagy is expanded at whatever point we are fasting while eating even modest quantities decrease it. Studies have shown that eating just 10g of fundamental amino acids (tracked down in excellent proteins) can turn off autophagy. A juice quick likely could be the response to give your body a decent 'spring clean' since juices are regularly exceptionally low in protein. Presently, autophagy and IGF-1 are two things that you neither need to be 'on' constantly or 'off' constantly. The key, as in many things, is tracking down the right equilibrium.

Fasting diminishes irritation
Irritation is a typical reaction to injury, pointed toward eliminating anything that's causing the injury and launching the recuperating system. However, a lot of them can be risky, just like the case in fiery circumstances like joint pain, atherosclerosis, and even dermatitis. Elevated degrees of muscle-to-fat

ratio are related to expansions in fiery markers like IL-6, TNFa, and CRP. Concentrates on a few different fasting designs show that these fiery markers will generally lessen during times of fasting. This is the situation for Ramadan (a day-to-day quick of 12-18 hours), a solitary day-to-day feast versus three dinners every day, and substitute day fasts. Intermittent fasting has been explicitly displayed to diminish the side effects of asthma, one more condition wherein an excess of irritation assumes a key part.

Fasting helps keep the heart and dissemination sound

Irritation is associated with cardiovascular illness, working together with elevated degrees of 'awful' fats in the blood. Most examinations on fasting show that they lessen fatty substance levels and work on the proportion of fatty substances to 'great' cholesterol (HDL - the vehicle protein that helps eliminate the abundance of cholesterol from the circulation system). In creature studies, protection from what is known as 'ischaemic injury' - the sort of corridor harm that is related to the development of plaques and solidifying of the veins, has been seen.

With everything taken into account, fasting appears to give the body an interior check-up and build protection from age-related diseases.

Fasting resets consistent eating

If you are somebody who eats constantly, you might have persistently high insulin levels. Insulin gives the sign to your body to store energy from your food with the goal that it very well may be gotten to later. It fundamentally acts by opening cells and permitting individual atoms of glucose to enter. It likewise advises the cells to make more protein and fat and to keep the current fat locked away inside.

This is completely planned to keep the degrees of glucose inside a firmly controlled range. Any sugar that isn't promptly needed for energy must be put away in the muscles or liver.

Elevated degrees of insulin in the body can expand the gamble of insulin obstruction (those locks get 'broken' and begin experiencing issues perceiving the 'key'.) After some time, insulin opposition builds the gamble of diabetes and has additionally been connected to cardiovascular illness, malignant growth, and other fiery ailments.

Eating "close to nothing and frequently", which is advanced by countless weight control plans, is tied in with keeping your body from delivering an excess of insulin on the double and just giving it the supplements that it can promptly put to utilise. However, to consume muscle versus fat, your insulin levels should be low.

In this way, if you eat pretty much nothing and frequently, your body will constantly be delivering a little insulin. Expanding the holes between dinners through fasting implies that you will get a spike in insulin after eating, then, at that point, a more extended timeframe where insulin isn't engaged in any way. The thought is that this won't just urge your body to consume fat, it will likewise assist with keeping up with its regular aversion to insulin.

Chapter 3

The missing key to a fruitful weight reduction

Getting thinner

Fruitful weight reduction doesn't expect individuals to follow a particular eating routine arrangement, for example, Thinning World or Atkins. All things considered, they ought to zero in on eating fewer calories and moving more to accomplish a negative energy balance.

Weight reduction is fundamentally reliant upon diminishing the absolute admission of calories, not changing the extent of sugar, fat, and protein in the eating regimen.

A sensible weight reduction objective to begin seeing medical advantages is a 5-10 percent decrease in body weight in more than 6 months.

A great many people can accomplish this objective by diminishing their complete calorie admission to someplace in the scope of 1,000-1,600 calories each day.

An eating routine of less than 1,000 calories each day won't give adequate day-to-day nourishment.

Following a half year of slimming down, the pace of weight reduction normally declines, and body weight keeps an eye on a level since individuals utilise less energy at a lower body weight. Following a weight support program of invigorating dietary patterns and ordinary active work is the most effective way to try not to recapture shed pounds.

Individuals who have a BMI equivalent to or higher than 30 with no stoutness-related medical issues might profit from assuming solution weight reduction meds. These could likewise be reasonable for individuals with a BMI equivalent to or higher than 27 with corpulence-related illnesses.

Nonetheless, an individual ought to just utilize drugs to help the above way of life change. If endeavors to shed pounds are ineffective and an individual's BMI arrives at 40 or over, careful treatment is a choice.

10 hints for effective weight reduction

People can get more fit and keep up with this misfortune by making a few reachable strides. These incorporate the accompanying:

1. Eat fluctuated, brilliant, healthfully thick food varieties.

Restorative dinners and bites ought to frame the underpinning of the human eating regimen. A basic method for making a dinner plan is to ensure that every feast comprises 50% foods grown from the ground, 25% entire grains, and 25 percent protein.

All out fibre admission ought to be 25-30 gramsTrusted Source (g) day to day.

Wipe out trans fats from the eating regimen, and limit the admission of immersed fats, which have areas of strength for the occurrence of coronary illness.

All things being equal, people can consume monounsaturated unsaturated fats (MUFA) or polyunsaturated unsaturated fats (PUFA), which are kinds of unsaturated fat.

The following food sources are fortifying and frequently wealthy in supplements:
*new products of the soil
*fish
*Vegetables
*nuts
*seeds
*entire grains, like earthy-coloured rice and cereal

Food sources not to eat include:
*food sources with added oils, spread, and sugar
*greasy red or handled meats
*prepared merchandise
*bagels
*white bread

*handled food sources

At times, eliminating specific food varieties from the eating regimen could make an individual lacking in a few fundamental nutrients and minerals. A nutritionist, dietitian, or another medical service proficient can encourage an individual to get an adequate number of supplements while they are following a health improvement plan.

2. Keep a food and weight journal
Self-observing is a basic variable in effectively getting thinner. Individuals can utilise a paper journal, versatile application, or committed site to record each thing of food that they devour every day. They can likewise gauge their advancement by recording their weight consistently.
The people who can follow their outcome in little augmentations and recognize actual changes are considerably more prone to adhere to a weight reduction routine.
Individuals can likewise monitor their weight record (BMI) by utilising a BMI mini-computer.

3.Take part in customary actual work and exercise

Customary active work can assist an individual with shedding pounds.

Customary activity is indispensable for both physical and psychological well-being. Expanding the recurrence of active work in a trained and deliberate manner is frequently significant for effective weight reduction.

One hour of moderate-force action each day, like lively strolling, is great. On the off chance that one hour out of each day is preposterous, the Mayo Facility recommends that an individual ought to hold back nothing of 150 minutes consistently.

Individuals who are not ordinarily truly dynamic ought to gradually build how much activity they do and steadily increment its force. This approach is the most manageable way for guaranteeing that ordinary activity turns into a piece of their way of life.

Similarly recording feasts can mentally assist with weight reduction, individuals may likewise profit from monitoring their active work. Many free portable applications are accessible that track an individual's calorie balance after they log their food admission and exercise.

On the off chance that the prospect of a full exercise appears to be threatening to somebody new to working out, they can start by doing the

accompanying exercises to expand their activity levels:
*using the stairwell
*raking leaves
*strolling a canine
*planting
*Moving
*playing open-air games
*stopping farther away from a structural entrance

People who have an okay of coronary illness are not going to require clinical evaluation in front of beginning an activity routine.

Nonetheless, an earlier clinical assessment might be fitting for certain individuals, incorporating those with diabetes. Any individual who is not certain about safe degrees of activity ought to address medical care proficiency.

4. Dispose of fluid calories
It is feasible to polish off many calories daily by drinking sugar-improved pop, tea, juice, or liquor. These are known as "void calories" since they give additional energy content without offering any nourishing advantages.

Except if an individual is drinking a smoothie to supplant a dinner, they ought to expect to adhere to water or unsweetened tea and espresso. Adding a sprinkle of new lemon or orange to the water can give flavour.

Try not to confuse parchedness with hunger. An individual can frequently fulfil sensations of craving between booked feast times with a beverage of water.

5. Measure servings and control segments

Eating a lot of any food, even low-calorie vegetables, can bring about weight gain.

Thus, individuals ought to abstain from assessing a serving size or eating food straightforwardly from the bundle. It is smarter to make use of estimating cups and serving size guides. Speculating prompts misjudging and the probability of eating a bigger than-needed segment.

The accompanying size examinations can help check food admission while eating out:

*A quarter of a cup is known as a golf ball

*one-half of a cup is a tennis ball

*1 cup is a baseball

*1 ounce (oz) of nuts is a free little bunch

*1 teaspoon is one playing bite the dust

*1 tablespoon is a thumb tip
*3 oz of meat is a deck of cards
*1 cut is a DVD

These sizes are not careful, however, they can help an individual with directing their food consumption when the right instruments are not free.

6. Eat carefully

Many people benefit from careful eating, which includes being completely mindful of why, how, when, where, and what they eat.

Settling on more curative food decisions is an immediate result of turning out to be more on top of the body.

People who practise careful eating additionally attempt to eat all the more leisurely and enjoy their food, focusing on the taste. Making dinner for 20 minutes permits the body to enrol every one of the signs of satiety.

It means a lot to zero in on being fulfilled after dinner as opposed to full and to remember that many "all regular" or low-fat food sources are not an empowering decision.

Individuals can likewise consider the accompanying inquiries concerning their dinner decision:

*Is it great "esteem" for the calorie cost?

*Will it give satiety?

*Are the fixings empowering?

*If it has a name, how much fat and sodium does it contain?

7. Upgrade and signal control

Numerous social and ecological prompts could empower superfluous eating. For instance, certain people are bound to gorge while staring at the TV. Others experience difficulty passing a bowl of treats to another individual without taking a piece.

By monitoring what might set out the craving to nibble on void calories, individuals can imagine ways of changing their daily schedule to restrict these triggers.

8. Prepare

Stocking up a kitchen with diet-accommodating food varieties and making organised feast plans will bring about more huge weight reduction.

Individuals hoping to get in shape or keep it off ought to get their kitchen free from handled or unhealthy foods and guarantee that they have the fixings available to simplify, refreshing dinners. Doing this can forestall fast, impromptu, and indiscreet eating.

Arranging food decisions before getting to get-togethers or cafés could likewise make the interaction more straightforward.

9. Look for social help

Taking the help of friends and family is a basic piece of an effective weight reduction venture.

Certain people might wish to welcome companions or relatives to go along with them, while others would like to utilise online entertainment to share their advancement.

Different roads of help might include:
*a positive informal organisation
*Gathering or individual advising

*Practice clubs or accomplices
*Representative help programs at work

10. Remain positive

Weight reduction is a progressive interaction, and an individual might feel deterred on the off chance that the pounds don't drop off at an incredible rate that they had expected.

Occasionally will be more diligent than others while adhering to a weight reduction or upkeep program. An effective health improvement plan requires the person to endure and not surrender when self-change appears to be excessively troublesome.

Certain individuals could have to reset their objectives, possibly by changing the all-out number of calories they are expecting to eat or changing their activity designs.

The significant thing is to keep an uplifting perspective and be determined to conquer the obstacles to effective weight reduction.

Chapter 4

A lady's approach to fasting

Discontinuous fasting has become progressively well-known as of late.

Dissimilar to most weight control plans that let you know what to eat, discontinuous fasting centres around when to eat by integrating customary transient diets into your daily practice.

This approach to eating might assist you with taking in fewer calories, getting in shape, and lowering your gamble of diabetes and coronary illness.

In any case, various examinations have recommended that irregular fasting may not be as helpful for ladies for what it's worth for men. Hence, ladies might have to follow a changed methodology.

What is irregular fasting?

Discontinuous fasting (IF) depicts an example of eating that cycles between times of fasting and ordinary eating.

The most widely recognized strategies are fasting for substitute days, every day 16-hour diets, or fasting for 24 hours, two days per week. With the end goal of this article, the term discontinuous fasting will be utilised to depict all regimens.

Not at all like most weight control plans, discontinuous fasting doesn't include following calories or macronutrients. There are no prerequisites about what food varieties to eat or keep away from, making it to a greater degree a way of life rather than an eating regimen.

Many individuals utilise discontinuous fasting to get fitter as it is a straightforward, helpful, and viable method for eating less and diminishing muscle versus fat.

It might likewise assist with decreasing the gamble of coronary illness and diabetes, safeguard bulk, and work on mental prosperity.

Additionally, this dietary example can assist with saving time in the kitchen as you have fewer dinners to design, plan, and cook.

Irregular Fasting Might Influence People In an unexpected way

There is some proof that irregular fasting may not be as useful for certain ladies for what it's worth for men.

One review showed that glucose control was demolished in ladies following three weeks of irregular fasting, which was not the situation in men.

There are likewise numerous narrative accounts of ladies who have encountered changes to their feminine cycles after beginning irregular fasting.

Such moves happen because female bodies are very delicate to calorie limitation.

At the point when calorie admission is low —, for example, from fasting for a long time or too habitually — a little piece of the cerebrum called the nerve centre is impacted.

This can upset the emission of gonadotropin-delivering chemical (GnRH), a chemical that helps discharge two conceptive chemicals: luteinizing chemical (LH) and follicle invigorating chemical.

At the point when these chemicals can't speak with the ovaries, you risk unpredictable periods, fruitlessness,

unfortunate bone well-being, and other well-being impacts.

Even though there are no equivalent human examinations, tests in rodents have shown that 3-6 months of substitute-day fasting caused a decrease in ovary size and sporadic regenerative cycles in female rodents.

Consequently, ladies ought to think about a changed way to deal with irregular fasting, like more limited fasting periods and fewer fasting days.

Best Sorts of Discontinuous Fasting for Ladies

With regards to eating less junk food, there is nobody size-fits-all methodology. This likewise applies to irregular fasting.

Ladies, as a rule, ought to adopt a more loosened-up strategy to fasting than men.

This might incorporate more limited fasting periods, fewer fasting days or potentially consuming few calories on the fasting days.

Here are the absolute best kinds of irregular fasting for ladies:

*Crescendo Technique: Fasting 12-16 hours for a few days every week. Fasting days ought to be nonconsecutive and separated equitably across the week (for instance, Monday, Wednesday, and Friday).

*Eat-stop-eat (likewise called the 24-hour convention): A 24-hour full quick more than once per week (limit of two times each week for ladies). Begin with 14-16 hour diets and bit by bit develop.

*The 5:2 Eating regimen (likewise called "The Quick Eating routine"): Confine calories to 25% of your typical intake (around 500 calories) for two days per week and eat "ordinarily" the other five days. Permit one day between fasting days.

*Changed Substitute Day Fasting: Fasting every other day yet eating "regularly" on non-fasting days. You are permitted to consume 20-25% of your typical calorie consumption (around 500 calories) on a fasting day.

*The 16/8 Strategy (likewise called the "Leangains technique"): Fasting for 16 hours per day and eating all calories inside an eight-hour window. Ladies are encouraged to begin with 14-hour diets and ultimately move toward 16 hours.

Whichever you pick, eating great during the non-fasting periods is as yet significant. On the off chance that you eat a lot of unfortunate, calorie-thick food varieties during the non-fasting time frames, you may not encounter similar weight reduction and medical advantages.

By the end of the day, the best methodology is one that you can endure and support in the long haul, and which brings about no bad wellbeing outcomes.

Security and Incidental Effects
Changed adaptations of discontinuous fasting seem, by all accounts, to be alright for most ladies.
That being said, various investigations have detailed a few incidental effects including hunger, state of mind swings, absence of focus, decreased energy, migraines, and terrible breath on fasting days.

There are likewise a few stories online of ladies who report that their feminine cycle halted while following an irregular fasting diet.

On the off chance that you have an ailment, you ought to talk with your primary care physician before attempting discontinuous fasting.

The clinical interview is especially significant for ladies who:

Have a past filled with dietary issues.

Have diabetes or consistently experience low glucose levels.

Are underweight, malnourished, or have healthful inadequacies?

Are pregnant, breastfeeding, or attempting to imagine?

Have ripeness issues or a past filled with amenorrhea (missed periods).

By the day's end, irregular fasting seems to have a decent wellbeing profile. However, assuming you experience any issues — such as loss of your monthly cycle — stop right away.

Chapter 5

instructions to construct a fasting way of life that will be reasonable for you

Fasting is an old food limitation technique that has become advocated for its many advantages to weight reduction, wellbeing and life span.

While conflicting with your body's signs to eat during a quick can feel unimaginable, we are as a matter of fact returning to the agrarian way of life that saw old people getting through long stretches of delayed fasting.

By the by, fasting stays a difficult dietary change that is hard to integrate into the bustling present day lifestyle. This guide can help you adjust and keep up with fasting in your way of life.

Various kinds of fasting

Caloric limitation offers various medical advantages, from weight reduction, assurance against infections including diabetes, cardiovascular illness and diseases and expanded life span - all through to the cycles of ketosis and autophagy.

There are different strategies to suit any way of life, from unconstrained feast skipping for those starting their fasting process, to outrageous 36-hour delayed diets.

A fair compromise can be tracked down in irregular fasting (IF), which switches back and forth between standard times of fasting and devouring and is particularly simple to adjust to occupied ways of life as it doesn't confine your eating routine during feast hours.

Discontinuous fasting comes in many structures: the 5:2 includes lessening your calorie consumption for two days seven days then, at that point, eating unhindered until the end of the week; the one dinner daily quick (OMAD), otherwise called the 'Fighter quick', includes just eating one colossal feast a day; while Time Confined Eating (TRE) comprises of day to day rotating windows of fasting and devouring.

Time Limited Eating (TRE) includes minimal responsibility as its fasting windows range from 12 hours with the short 12:12 quick, to 20 hours with the difficult 20:4 quick.

The 16:8 is one the most famous types of TRE that follows the body's normal circadian mood, consisting of 8 hours of devouring during the day followed by 16 hours of fasting for the time being. A great many people total some type of quick for the time being since it is genuinely difficult to eat while you are resting!

This implies you can undoubtedly accomplish the 16:8 by broadening this regular quick by a couple of hours in the first part of the day and night. While outrageous delayed diets are best kept away from fledglings, explore different avenues regarding different fasting techniques until you find the one that fits impeccably into your way of life.

Defining sensible objectives

Not at all like trend eats less, caloric limitation is an economical weight reduction strategy that works over the long haul by setting the body under supplement pressure, setting off the metabolic course of ketosis (fat consuming).

Be that as it may, it is feasible to get out of hand and put a lot of weight on the body, causing exhaustion and mental strain and fixing fasting benefits. For instance, holding back nothing hour quick for a speedy weight reduction fix as a fledgling might prompt unfriendly incidental effects.

All things considered, adjust your quick to your drawn out weight reduction objectives while staying sensible. Set little, continuous irregular fasting objectives that are more effectively reachable than inconceivable delayed fasting.

For instance, a week by week 12-hour quick is a superior split the difference. After your most memorable seven day stretch of fasting, increment your fasting window or recurrence each succeeding week until you arrive at a level that you are OK with.

At this point, you may currently be content with the weight reduction results accomplished by more limited diets and on the off chance that not, your body will be more ready to get through delayed fasting.

The most effective method to abstain from eating during fasting

Until your body becomes used to caloric limitation, it is not difficult to become distracted with the prospect of food. Fortunately, there are a few methodologies to stay away from this, the key being planning.

Record your standard timetable as well as any occasions that, right off the bat, include eating, fitting fasting in the hours around this to guarantee that your public activity doesn't disturb your quick as well as the other way around

Taking into account that most human holding rotates around eating, timing your quick around your public activity permits you to remain focused on both your quick and your companions.

Arranging a basic food item rundown and cooking timetable can assist you with having solid, satisfying dinners prepared for when you break your quick

One more method for planning for fasting is by eating soundly before your quick or during the devouring hours of a discontinuous quick.

Wiping out or limiting admission of sugars and refined carbs normal in desserts, soda pops and white bread before a quick is useful as these food varieties adversely influence how the body processes fat.

All things being equal, select the exemplary Mediterranean eating regimen with the ideal equilibrium of sound fats from olive oil, protein from fish and low glycaemic sugars from vegetables and entire grains to praise your picked quick. This will likewise assist you with feeling more full for longer utilising less caloric admission.

Permit yourself a periodic extravagance by integrating your number one dinners and snacks into your devouring hours on the off chance that it makes you more roused to stay devoted to your quick - all with some restraint obviously.

It is critical to try not to indulge during the periods when you can eat. Over-making up for fasting periods by eating huge, unhealthy dinners during devouring periods can leave you feeling dormant as the body goes through energy to process the abrupt renewed introduction of food.

Overseeing segment sizes will assist you with staying in command over your eating, and rehearsing irregular fasting might actually assist with lessening hunger.

Taking into account that individuals will more often than not eat undesirable food sources in more noteworthy sums when they are exhausted as an interruption, it is essential to stay occupied while fasting.

For instance, expanding your work-out daily schedule during caloric limitation supports the medical advantages of your quick as well as keeping your psyche and body involved and away from food desires.

While demanding activity while fasting isn't suggested, light oxygen consuming exercises like strolling and yoga or strength-based exercises for a limit of one hour out of each day are great. Consolidating another activity system or side interest close by your quick will divert you from eating as well as assist you with accomplishing all encompassing wellbeing.

At long last, share your caloric limitation objectives with others as they can assist with holding you under tight restraints and proposition uplifting statements, be it family or work partners relying upon the hour of day your quick falls.

This will consider you more responsible to your weight reduction objectives, and seeing you contact them might try and switch others over completely to the fasting way of life!

On the other hand, specific applications like the life span application Mankind are accessible to monitor your quick all day, every day.

This can help you put forth and picture objectives, remind you to eat or quick with alerts and give wholesome counsel, successfully gamifying your quick and making it more enjoyable to finish.

Chapter 6

food sources that help your chemicals

Chemicals are little particles that go about as compound couriers in the human body. They are delivered by the endocrine organs and travel all through the circulatory system following up on cells, organs, and tissue to apply a particular impact.
Food varieties that might assist with adjusting chemicals

Offsetting chemicals with medications can be troublesome. Meds endorsed by specialists are suitable for select ladies who have an extremely hormonal awkward nature. Most ladies, nonetheless, don't need such escalated treatment for their hormonal dysregulation. These ladies can utilize food varieties that assist the body with making the required chemicals normally.

We should take a gander at the food sources known to assist with working on hormonal dysregulation and equilibrium chemicals normally:

*Flaxseeds.

Flaxseeds seem to have benefits for ladies with PCOS. Taking flaxseeds advances further developed metabolic boundaries that outcome in additional weight reduction and further developed fruitfulness.

*Broccoli.

Broccoli and different individuals from the Brassica family are known to advance upgraded liver well-being and diminish the possibility of having metabolic liver sickness. This can assist ladies with PCOS to balance their chemicals. Moreover, eating broccoli can assist with reestablishing the stomach microbiome, which works on metabolic well-being.

*Avocados.

Avocados are an astounding wellspring of monounsaturated fats. They can bring down cholesterol and fatty oils, diminishing your gamble of coronary illness. They can help in lessening aggravation and permit you to fabricate chemicals.

* Salmon.

Salmon is a fantastic wellspring of omega-3 unsaturated fats, fundamental for some parts of well-being. The protein in salmon and other low-mercury fish upgrades satiety and doesn't cause glucose changes.

*Quinoa.
Quinoa can adjust chemicals by diminishing glucose, further developing the lipid profile, and decreasing gut fat. These are significant impacts that might further develop PCOS side effects and results.

*Spinach.
Spinach and other salad greens give a wide exhibit of phytonutrients. When eaten routinely by ladies with PCOS, spinach can diminish midsection fat and work on the metabolic profile, prompting improved chemical equilibrium.

*Almonds.
Almonds are a superb nibble choice for ladies. They stifle cravings and diminish glucose vacillations without adding to weight gain.

*Chia seeds.

Chia seeds are brilliant wellsprings of fibre since they leak water, taking into consideration improved GI capability. At the point when you eat them, they might make a mitigating difference and could upgrade circulatory strain guidelines. Chia seeds are likewise useful in lessening wide swings in glucose.

*Turkey.

Turkey contains tryptophan, which is an amino corrosive forerunner in the development of a few significant states of mind and craving synapses. At the point when these synapses are adjusted, you might have further developed rest and decreased nibbling.

*Blueberries.

Blueberries are high in cancer prevention agents, which diminish the weight of the cells. They have been displayed to improve female and male fruitfulness.

*Olive oil.

Olive oil is stacked with polyunsaturated fats that assist in bringing down irritation and decrease midsection fat. It has been demonstrated to be harmful to bosom malignant growth cells, which might imply that it further develops the chemical offset for ladies with oestrogen-delicate tumours like bosom disease.

*Lentils.

Lentils are high in fibre and an amazing wellspring of starch. They diminish glucose variances, lower gut fat substance, and safeguard the stomach microbiome. These can assist with reestablishing your body's regular chemical levels.

*Greek yoghourt.

Yogurt is a mature food that contains sound probiotics. This expands your stomach microbiome and takes into consideration normal chemical remaking.

*Green tea.

Green tea is high in cancer prevention agents, and that implies it supports boosting cell well-being. For ladies with PCOS, green tea can lessen insulin opposition and may assist with upgrading digestion.

*Pomegranates.
These are high in cancer prevention agents and safeguard against high glucose and paunch fat. They can be useful in rectifying the fiery states that forestall ordinary hormonal equilibrium.

*Eggs.
Eggs are a great wellspring of protein and contain choline for cerebrum wellbeing. Eggs additionally smother hunger and add to weight reduction by saving you more full for longer.

*Tofu.
Soy isoflavones are a significant part of tofu. They assist with adjusting female chemicals in menopausal ladies and advance decreased muscle versus fat levels as they contain almost no additional fat. This by itself can assist ladies with PCOS to have more adjusted chemical levels.

*Aged food varieties.
Aged food varieties like yoghourt, miso, tempeh, sauerkraut, and kimchi add solid probiotics to

augment your stomach's well-being. Great stomach well-being implies less aggravation and works on hormonal levels.

*Cinnamon.
Cinnamon comes in a few kinds. Most contain coumarin which adds to its mitigating properties. It balances out glucose, advances decreased muscle-to-fat ratio, and lessens lipid levels.

As a rule, when irritation is decreased, you will have a more ideal climate for lessening the weight on the cells of your body. This permits your chemicals to adjust normally. In ladies with PCOS, a diminished muscle-to-fat ratio implies further developed chemical levels and fewer side effects.

While most food varieties are protected to eat with some restraint, the food varieties to help your particular condition may not be similar ones to assist someone else with comparable issues. Since adjusting chemicals utilising food is some of the time complex, you would profit from the counsel of your medical services supplier or a chemical well-being nutritionist to assist you with dealing with your special conditions.

Chapter 7

instructions to break your fasting

At the point when you're prepared to break a quick, centre around effectively endured food sources that don't contain high measures of sugar, fat, fibre, or complex carbs that could be hard to process. You can then move once more into an ordinary, smart dieting design.

What to Eat While Breaking a Short Quick
While there is less to consider while you're breaking a quick that you've been on for under 24 hours, you ought to in any case focus on your most memorable dinner of the day to receive the greatest rewards of fasting. You will be substantially more delicate to starches in the wake of fasting, so eating bigger measures of these food varieties might expand your gamble for a glucose spike.

Instructions to Break Your Quick
1A great guideline is to zero in on protein first in the wake of fasting to advance a more modest glycemic reaction. From that point, you can partake in some

low glycemic carbs and solid fats in your primary dinner, preferably around 30 after an hour. For instance, some lean protein like turkey or a whey protein shake are great choices.

Food sources like bread, bagels, and cereal, will commonly make glucose spike rapidly in the wake of fasting and may cause an "energy crash," advancing more sensations of craving and laziness over the day. However, you ought to attempt to eat most sugars during sunshine hours to line up with your circadian rhythms, the sort of starches you eat, and what you pair them with issues. Picking complex, fiber-rich sugars that are low in the glycemic record is a decent decision here. Always think avocado, berries, flaxseed, chia seeds, steel-cut oats, and squash.

Segment Size Matters
Also, shouldn't something be said about segment size? That matters as well. On the off chance that you eat an enormous feast since you're truly ravenous falling off your quick, attempt to have a little part first, find out how you feel satiety-wise, and afterward turn out for seconds assuming you're as yet eager. Eating a lot excessively fast can cause

stomach-related trouble or swelling, so eating gradually and carefully here is smart.

Some example dinners for breaking a short quick:
A piece of cheddar 15 minutes before eating steel-cut oats with protein powder, nuts, and berries.One hard-bubbled egg 15 minutes before eating a feast like salmon, steamed vegetables, avocado, and feta.One or two bits of cut turkey 15 minutes before eating unsweetened Greek yogurt with berries, nuts, and chia seeds.

What to Eat While Breaking a Drawn-out Quick
A drawn-out quick is the point at which you've been fasting for 24 hours or more, and getting over it can be precarious. A little foundation on what's going on in your body falling off of a quick: following 24 hours of fasting, a great many people's glycogen (put away glucose) stores have been fundamentally exhausted. Your body then, at that point, starts to consume and put away fat for energy. Your body separates fat through lipolysis, making free unsaturated fats enter your circulation system and be used for fuel through beta-oxidation and ketone body arrangement. Between 24-72 hours of fasting, ketone bodies become your body's essential energy

source. Furthermore, the body makes new glucose from glycerol and amino acids through gluconeogenesis to supply the cerebrum and red platelets with glucose.

Your Craving Chemicals

All in all, what ends up wanting?
That's what one review showed even though ghrelin rises and falls in a cyclic example connected with your circadian musicality, all-out ghrelin levels decline like clockwork of fasting. Along these lines, by day three, generally ghrelin yield was lower than on days one and two. These outcomes might make sense of why generally speaking yearning levels appear to diminish around the third day of a quick. Ghrelin sets off your stomach's parietal cells to begin discharging the stomach-related squeezes and stomach corrosive we want to separate approaching food.